3 APPLE A DAY DIET

TRACK YOUR WEIGHT LOSS PROGRESS
WITH CALORIE COUNTING CHART

Copyright 2015

How many calories ?

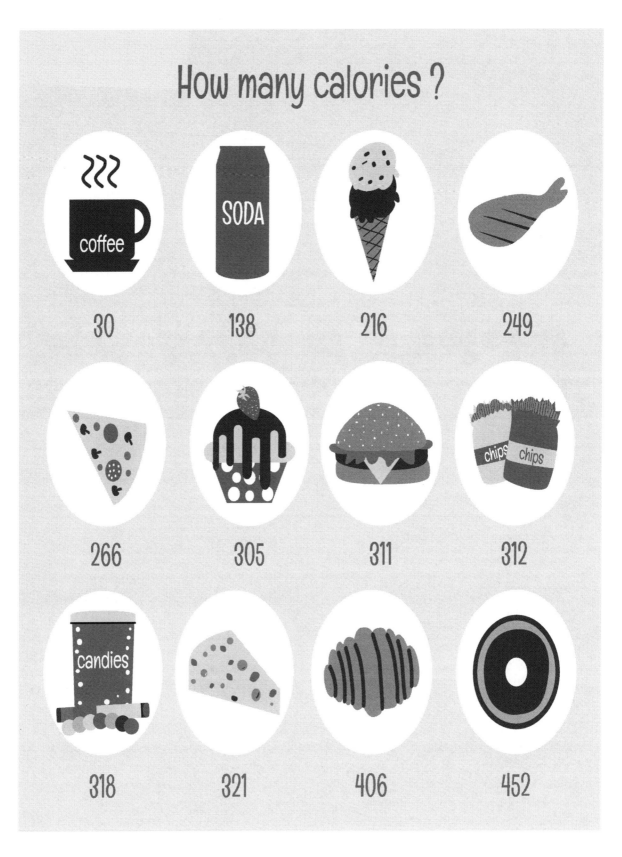

DATE:

BREAKFAST

DESCRIPTION	QTY	PROTEINS	VEGGIES	FRUITS & NUTS	CARBS	FATS

LUNCH

DESCRIPTION	QTY	PROTEINS	VEGGIES	FRUITS & NUTS	CARBS	FATS

DINNER

DESCRIPTION	QTY	PROTEINS	VEGGIES	FRUITS & NUTS	CARBS	FATS

SNACKS

NOTES:

_____

_____

_____

_____

_____

_____

DATE:

BREAKFAST

DESCRIPTION	QTY	PROTEINS	VEGGIES	FRUITS & NUTS	CARBS	FATS

LUNCH

DESCRIPTION	QTY	PROTEINS	VEGGIES	FRUITS & NUTS	CARBS	FATS

DINNER

DESCRIPTION	QTY	PROTEINS	VEGGIES	FRUITS & NUTS	CARBS	FATS

SNACKS

NOTES:

_____

_____

_____

_____

_____

_____

DATE:

BREAKFAST

DESCRIPTION	QTY	PROTEINS	VEGGIES	FRUITS & NUTS	CARBS	FATS

LUNCH

DESCRIPTION	QTY	PROTEINS	VEGGIES	FRUITS & NUTS	CARBS	FATS

DINNER

DESCRIPTION	QTY	PROTEINS	VEGGIES	FRUITS & NUTS	CARBS	FATS

SNACKS

NOTES:

_____

_____

_____

_____

_____

_____

DATE:

BREAKFAST

DESCRIPTION	QTY	PROTEINS	VEGGIES	FRUITS & NUTS	CARBS	FATS

LUNCH

DESCRIPTION	QTY	PROTEINS	VEGGIES	FRUITS & NUTS	CARBS	FATS

DINNER

DESCRIPTION	QTY	PROTEINS	VEGGIES	FRUITS & NUTS	CARBS	FATS

SNACKS

NOTES:

_____

_____

_____

_____

_____

_____

DATE:

BREAKFAST

DESCRIPTION	QTY	PROTEINS	VEGGIES	FRUITS & NUTS	CARBS	FATS

LUNCH

DESCRIPTION	QTY	PROTEINS	VEGGIES	FRUITS & NUTS	CARBS	FATS

DINNER

DESCRIPTION	QTY	PROTEINS	VEGGIES	FRUITS & NUTS	CARBS	FATS

SNACKS

NOTES:

DATE:

BREAKFAST

DESCRIPTION	QTY	PROTEINS	VEGGIES	FRUITS & NUTS	CARBS	FATS

LUNCH

DESCRIPTION	QTY	PROTEINS	VEGGIES	FRUITS & NUTS	CARBS	FATS

DINNER

DESCRIPTION	QTY	PROTEINS	VEGGIES	FRUITS & NUTS	CARBS	FATS

SNACKS

NOTES:

_____

_____

_____

_____

_____

_____

DATE:

BREAKFAST

DESCRIPTION	QTY	PROTEINS	VEGGIES	FRUITS & NUTS	CARBS	FATS

LUNCH

DESCRIPTION	QTY	PROTEINS	VEGGIES	FRUITS & NUTS	CARBS	FATS

DINNER

DESCRIPTION	QTY	PROTEINS	VEGGIES	FRUITS & NUTS	CARBS	FATS

SNACKS

NOTES:

DATE:

BREAKFAST

DESCRIPTION	QTY	PROTEINS	VEGGIES	FRUITS & NUTS	CARBS	FATS

LUNCH

DESCRIPTION	QTY	PROTEINS	VEGGIES	FRUITS & NUTS	CARBS	FATS

DINNER

DESCRIPTION	QTY	PROTEINS	VEGGIES	FRUITS & NUTS	CARBS	FATS

SNACKS

NOTES:

DATE:

BREAKFAST

DESCRIPTION	QTY	PROTEINS	VEGGIES	FRUITS & NUTS	CARBS	FATS

LUNCH

DESCRIPTION	QTY	PROTEINS	VEGGIES	FRUITS & NUTS	CARBS	FATS

DINNER

DESCRIPTION	QTY	PROTEINS	VEGGIES	FRUITS & NUTS	CARBS	FATS

SNACKS

NOTES:

DATE:

BREAKFAST

DESCRIPTION	QTY	PROTEINS	VEGGIES	FRUITS & NUTS	CARBS	FATS

LUNCH

DESCRIPTION	QTY	PROTEINS	VEGGIES	FRUITS & NUTS	CARBS	FATS

DINNER

DESCRIPTION	QTY	PROTEINS	VEGGIES	FRUITS & NUTS	CARBS	FATS

SNACKS

NOTES:

DATE:

BREAKFAST

DESCRIPTION	QTY	PROTEINS	VEGGIES	FRUITS & NUTS	CARBS	FATS

LUNCH

DESCRIPTION	QTY	PROTEINS	VEGGIES	FRUITS & NUTS	CARBS	FATS

DINNER

DESCRIPTION	QTY	PROTEINS	VEGGIES	FRUITS & NUTS	CARBS	FATS

SNACKS

NOTES:

DATE:

BREAKFAST

DESCRIPTION	QTY	PROTEINS	VEGGIES	FRUITS & NUTS	CARBS	FATS

LUNCH

DESCRIPTION	QTY	PROTEINS	VEGGIES	FRUITS & NUTS	CARBS	FATS

DINNER

DESCRIPTION	QTY	PROTEINS	VEGGIES	FRUITS & NUTS	CARBS	FATS

SNACKS

NOTES:

_____

_____

_____

_____

_____

_____

DATE:

BREAKFAST

DESCRIPTION	QTY	PROTEINS	VEGGIES	FRUITS & NUTS	CARBS	FATS

LUNCH

DESCRIPTION	QTY	PROTEINS	VEGGIES	FRUITS & NUTS	CARBS	FATS

DINNER

DESCRIPTION	QTY	PROTEINS	VEGGIES	FRUITS & NUTS	CARBS	FATS

SNACKS

NOTES:

DATE:

BREAKFAST

DESCRIPTION	QTY	PROTEINS	VEGGIES	FRUITS & NUTS	CARBS	FATS

LUNCH

DESCRIPTION	QTY	PROTEINS	VEGGIES	FRUITS & NUTS	CARBS	FATS

DINNER

DESCRIPTION	QTY	PROTEINS	VEGGIES	FRUITS & NUTS	CARBS	FATS

SNACKS

NOTES:

_____

_____

_____

_____

_____

_____

_____

DATE:

BREAKFAST

DESCRIPTION	QTY	PROTEINS	VEGGIES	FRUITS & NUTS	CARBS	FATS

LUNCH

DESCRIPTION	QTY	PROTEINS	VEGGIES	FRUITS & NUTS	CARBS	FATS

DINNER

DESCRIPTION	QTY	PROTEINS	VEGGIES	FRUITS & NUTS	CARBS	FATS

SNACKS

NOTES:

DATE:

BREAKFAST

DESCRIPTION	QTY	PROTEINS	VEGGIES	FRUITS & NUTS	CARBS	FATS

LUNCH

DESCRIPTION	QTY	PROTEINS	VEGGIES	FRUITS & NUTS	CARBS	FATS

DINNER

DESCRIPTION	QTY	PROTEINS	VEGGIES	FRUITS & NUTS	CARBS	FATS

SNACKS

NOTES:

_____

_____

_____

_____

_____

_____

_____

DATE:

BREAKFAST

DESCRIPTION	QTY	PROTEINS	VEGGIES	FRUITS & NUTS	CARBS	FATS

LUNCH

DESCRIPTION	QTY	PROTEINS	VEGGIES	FRUITS & NUTS	CARBS	FATS

DINNER

DESCRIPTION	QTY	PROTEINS	VEGGIES	FRUITS & NUTS	CARBS	FATS

SNACKS

NOTES:

_____

_____

_____

_____

_____

_____

DATE:

BREAKFAST

DESCRIPTION	QTY	PROTEINS	VEGGIES	FRUITS & NUTS	CARBS	FATS

LUNCH

DESCRIPTION	QTY	PROTEINS	VEGGIES	FRUITS & NUTS	CARBS	FATS

DINNER

DESCRIPTION	QTY	PROTEINS	VEGGIES	FRUITS & NUTS	CARBS	FATS

SNACKS

NOTES:

_____

_____

_____

_____

_____

_____

DATE:

BREAKFAST

DESCRIPTION	QTY	PROTEINS	VEGGIES	FRUITS & NUTS	CARBS	FATS

LUNCH

DESCRIPTION	QTY	PROTEINS	VEGGIES	FRUITS & NUTS	CARBS	FATS

DINNER

DESCRIPTION	QTY	PROTEINS	VEGGIES	FRUITS & NUTS	CARBS	FATS

SNACKS

NOTES:

_____

_____

_____

_____

_____

_____

DATE:

BREAKFAST

DESCRIPTION	QTY	PROTEINS	VEGGIES	FRUITS & NUTS	CARBS	FATS

LUNCH

DESCRIPTION	QTY	PROTEINS	VEGGIES	FRUITS & NUTS	CARBS	FATS

DINNER

DESCRIPTION	QTY	PROTEINS	VEGGIES	FRUITS & NUTS	CARBS	FATS

SNACKS

NOTES:

_____

_____

_____

_____

_____

_____

DATE:

BREAKFAST

DESCRIPTION	QTY	PROTEINS	VEGGIES	FRUITS & NUTS	CARBS	FATS

LUNCH

DESCRIPTION	QTY	PROTEINS	VEGGIES	FRUITS & NUTS	CARBS	FATS

DINNER

DESCRIPTION	QTY	PROTEINS	VEGGIES	FRUITS & NUTS	CARBS	FATS

SNACKS

NOTES:

_____

_____

_____

_____

_____

_____

_____

DATE:

BREAKFAST

DESCRIPTION	QTY	PROTEINS	VEGGIES	FRUITS & NUTS	CARBS	FATS

LUNCH

DESCRIPTION	QTY	PROTEINS	VEGGIES	FRUITS & NUTS	CARBS	FATS

DINNER

DESCRIPTION	QTY	PROTEINS	VEGGIES	FRUITS & NUTS	CARBS	FATS

SNACKS

NOTES:

DATE:

BREAKFAST

DESCRIPTION	QTY	PROTEINS	VEGGIES	FRUITS & NUTS	CARBS	FATS

LUNCH

DESCRIPTION	QTY	PROTEINS	VEGGIES	FRUITS & NUTS	CARBS	FATS

DINNER

DESCRIPTION	QTY	PROTEINS	VEGGIES	FRUITS & NUTS	CARBS	FATS

SNACKS

NOTES:

_____

_____

_____

_____

_____

_____

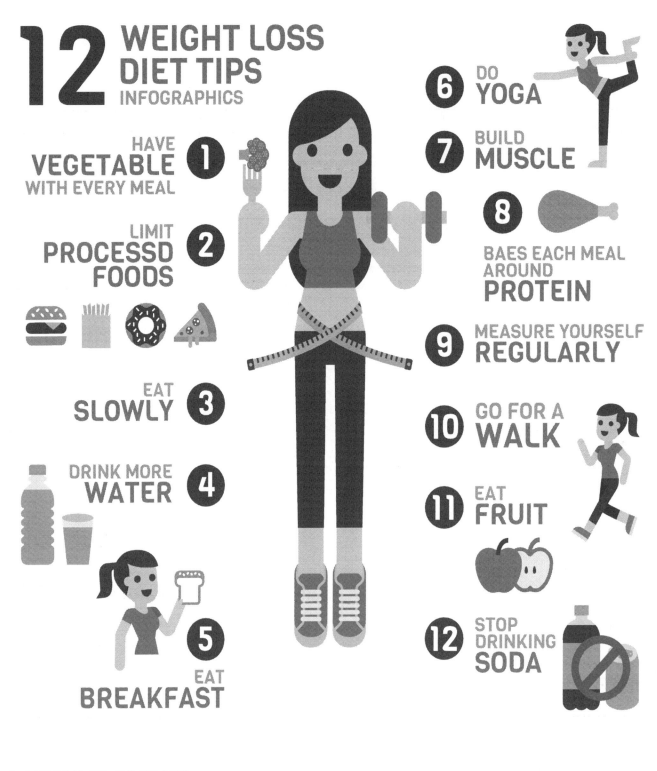

12 WEIGHT LOSS DIET TIPS
INFOGRAPHICS

HAVE **1** **VEGETABLE** WITH EVERY MEAL

LIMIT **2** **PROCESSD FOODS**

EAT **3** **SLOWLY**

DRINK MORE **4** **WATER**

5 EAT **BREAKFAST**

6 DO **YOGA**

7 BUILD **MUSCLE**

8 BAES EACH MEAL AROUND **PROTEIN**

9 MEASURE YOURSELF **REGULARLY**

10 GO FOR A **WALK**

11 EAT **FRUIT**

12 STOP DRINKING **SODA**

DAILY REMINDER:

_____

_____

_____

_____

DATE:

BREAKFAST

DESCRIPTION	QTY	PROTEINS	VEGGIES	FRUITS & NUTS	CARBS	FATS

LUNCH

DESCRIPTION	QTY	PROTEINS	VEGGIES	FRUITS & NUTS	CARBS	FATS

DINNER

DESCRIPTION	QTY	PROTEINS	VEGGIES	FRUITS & NUTS	CARBS	FATS

SNACKS

NOTES:

DATE:

BREAKFAST

DESCRIPTION	QTY	PROTEINS	VEGGIES	FRUITS & NUTS	CARBS	FATS

LUNCH

DESCRIPTION	QTY	PROTEINS	VEGGIES	FRUITS & NUTS	CARBS	FATS

DINNER

DESCRIPTION	QTY	PROTEINS	VEGGIES	FRUITS & NUTS	CARBS	FATS

SNACKS

NOTES:

_____

_____

_____

_____

_____

_____

DATE:

BREAKFAST

DESCRIPTION	QTY	PROTEINS	VEGGIES	FRUITS & NUTS	CARBS	FATS

LUNCH

DESCRIPTION	QTY	PROTEINS	VEGGIES	FRUITS & NUTS	CARBS	FATS

DINNER

DESCRIPTION	QTY	PROTEINS	VEGGIES	FRUITS & NUTS	CARBS	FATS

SNACKS

NOTES:

_____

_____

_____

_____

_____

_____

_____

DATE:

BREAKFAST

DESCRIPTION	QTY	PROTEINS	VEGGIES	FRUITS & NUTS	CARBS	FATS

LUNCH

DESCRIPTION	QTY	PROTEINS	VEGGIES	FRUITS & NUTS	CARBS	FATS

DINNER

DESCRIPTION	QTY	PROTEINS	VEGGIES	FRUITS & NUTS	CARBS	FATS

SNACKS

NOTES:

DATE:

BREAKFAST

DESCRIPTION	QTY	PROTEINS	VEGGIES	FRUITS & NUTS	CARBS	FATS

LUNCH

DESCRIPTION	QTY	PROTEINS	VEGGIES	FRUITS & NUTS	CARBS	FATS

DINNER

DESCRIPTION	QTY	PROTEINS	VEGGIES	FRUITS & NUTS	CARBS	FATS

SNACKS

NOTES:

DATE:

BREAKFAST

DESCRIPTION	QTY	PROTEINS	VEGGIES	FRUITS & NUTS	CARBS	FATS

LUNCH

DESCRIPTION	QTY	PROTEINS	VEGGIES	FRUITS & NUTS	CARBS	FATS

DINNER

DESCRIPTION	QTY	PROTEINS	VEGGIES	FRUITS & NUTS	CARBS	FATS

SNACKS

NOTES:

_____

_____

_____

_____

_____

_____

DATE:

BREAKFAST

DESCRIPTION	QTY	PROTEINS	VEGGIES	FRUITS & NUTS	CARBS	FATS

LUNCH

DESCRIPTION	QTY	PROTEINS	VEGGIES	FRUITS & NUTS	CARBS	FATS

DINNER

DESCRIPTION	QTY	PROTEINS	VEGGIES	FRUITS & NUTS	CARBS	FATS

SNACKS

NOTES:

_____

_____

_____

_____

_____

_____

DATE:

BREAKFAST

DESCRIPTION	QTY	PROTEINS	VEGGIES	FRUITS & NUTS	CARBS	FATS

LUNCH

DESCRIPTION	QTY	PROTEINS	VEGGIES	FRUITS & NUTS	CARBS	FATS

DINNER

DESCRIPTION	QTY	PROTEINS	VEGGIES	FRUITS & NUTS	CARBS	FATS

SNACKS

NOTES:

DATE:

BREAKFAST

DESCRIPTION	QTY	PROTEINS	VEGGIES	FRUITS & NUTS	CARBS	FATS

LUNCH

DESCRIPTION	QTY	PROTEINS	VEGGIES	FRUITS & NUTS	CARBS	FATS

DINNER

DESCRIPTION	QTY	PROTEINS	VEGGIES	FRUITS & NUTS	CARBS	FATS

SNACKS

NOTES:

_____

_____

_____

_____

_____

_____

DATE:

BREAKFAST

DESCRIPTION	QTY	PROTEINS	VEGGIES	FRUITS & NUTS	CARBS	FATS

LUNCH

DESCRIPTION	QTY	PROTEINS	VEGGIES	FRUITS & NUTS	CARBS	FATS

DINNER

DESCRIPTION	QTY	PROTEINS	VEGGIES	FRUITS & NUTS	CARBS	FATS

SNACKS

NOTES:

DATE:

BREAKFAST

DESCRIPTION	QTY	PROTEINS	VEGGIES	FRUITS & NUTS	CARBS	FATS

LUNCH

DESCRIPTION	QTY	PROTEINS	VEGGIES	FRUITS & NUTS	CARBS	FATS

DINNER

DESCRIPTION	QTY	PROTEINS	VEGGIES	FRUITS & NUTS	CARBS	FATS

SNACKS

NOTES:

_____

_____

_____

_____

_____

_____

DATE:

BREAKFAST

DESCRIPTION	QTY	PROTEINS	VEGGIES	FRUITS & NUTS	CARBS	FATS

LUNCH

DESCRIPTION	QTY	PROTEINS	VEGGIES	FRUITS & NUTS	CARBS	FATS

DINNER

DESCRIPTION	QTY	PROTEINS	VEGGIES	FRUITS & NUTS	CARBS	FATS

SNACKS

NOTES:

DATE:

BREAKFAST

DESCRIPTION	QTY	PROTEINS	VEGGIES	FRUITS & NUTS	CARBS	FATS

LUNCH

DESCRIPTION	QTY	PROTEINS	VEGGIES	FRUITS & NUTS	CARBS	FATS

DINNER

DESCRIPTION	QTY	PROTEINS	VEGGIES	FRUITS & NUTS	CARBS	FATS

SNACKS

NOTES:

_____

_____

_____

_____

_____

_____

DATE:

BREAKFAST

DESCRIPTION	QTY	PROTEINS	VEGGIES	FRUITS & NUTS	CARBS	FATS

LUNCH

DESCRIPTION	QTY	PROTEINS	VEGGIES	FRUITS & NUTS	CARBS	FATS

DINNER

DESCRIPTION	QTY	PROTEINS	VEGGIES	FRUITS & NUTS	CARBS	FATS

SNACKS

NOTES:

_____

_____

_____

_____

_____

_____

DATE:

BREAKFAST

DESCRIPTION	QTY	PROTEINS	VEGGIES	FRUITS & NUTS	CARBS	FATS

LUNCH

DESCRIPTION	QTY	PROTEINS	VEGGIES	FRUITS & NUTS	CARBS	FATS

DINNER

DESCRIPTION	QTY	PROTEINS	VEGGIES	FRUITS & NUTS	CARBS	FATS

SNACKS

NOTES:

DATE:

BREAKFAST

DESCRIPTION	QTY	PROTEINS	VEGGIES	FRUITS & NUTS	CARBS	FATS

LUNCH

DESCRIPTION	QTY	PROTEINS	VEGGIES	FRUITS & NUTS	CARBS	FATS

DINNER

DESCRIPTION	QTY	PROTEINS	VEGGIES	FRUITS & NUTS	CARBS	FATS

SNACKS

NOTES:

DATE:

BREAKFAST

DESCRIPTION	QTY	PROTEINS	VEGGIES	FRUITS & NUTS	CARBS	FATS

LUNCH

DESCRIPTION	QTY	PROTEINS	VEGGIES	FRUITS & NUTS	CARBS	FATS

DINNER

DESCRIPTION	QTY	PROTEINS	VEGGIES	FRUITS & NUTS	CARBS	FATS

SNACKS

NOTES:

DATE:

BREAKFAST

DESCRIPTION	QTY	PROTEINS	VEGGIES	FRUITS & NUTS	CARBS	FATS

LUNCH

DESCRIPTION	QTY	PROTEINS	VEGGIES	FRUITS & NUTS	CARBS	FATS

DINNER

DESCRIPTION	QTY	PROTEINS	VEGGIES	FRUITS & NUTS	CARBS	FATS

SNACKS

NOTES:

_____

_____

_____

_____

_____

_____

DATE:

BREAKFAST

DESCRIPTION	QTY	PROTEINS	VEGGIES	FRUITS & NUTS	CARBS	FATS

LUNCH

DESCRIPTION	QTY	PROTEINS	VEGGIES	FRUITS & NUTS	CARBS	FATS

DINNER

DESCRIPTION	QTY	PROTEINS	VEGGIES	FRUITS & NUTS	CARBS	FATS

SNACKS

NOTES:

_____

_____

_____

_____

_____

_____

DATE:

BREAKFAST

DESCRIPTION	QTY	PROTEINS	VEGGIES	FRUITS & NUTS	CARBS	FATS

LUNCH

DESCRIPTION	QTY	PROTEINS	VEGGIES	FRUITS & NUTS	CARBS	FATS

DINNER

DESCRIPTION	QTY	PROTEINS	VEGGIES	FRUITS & NUTS	CARBS	FATS

SNACKS

NOTES:

DATE:

BREAKFAST

DESCRIPTION	QTY	PROTEINS	VEGGIES	FRUITS & NUTS	CARBS	FATS

LUNCH

DESCRIPTION	QTY	PROTEINS	VEGGIES	FRUITS & NUTS	CARBS	FATS

DINNER

DESCRIPTION	QTY	PROTEINS	VEGGIES	FRUITS & NUTS	CARBS	FATS

SNACKS

NOTES:

_____

_____

_____

_____

_____

_____

DATE:

BREAKFAST

DESCRIPTION	QTY	PROTEINS	VEGGIES	FRUITS & NUTS	CARBS	FATS

LUNCH

DESCRIPTION	QTY	PROTEINS	VEGGIES	FRUITS & NUTS	CARBS	FATS

DINNER

DESCRIPTION	QTY	PROTEINS	VEGGIES	FRUITS & NUTS	CARBS	FATS

SNACKS

NOTES:

DATE:

BREAKFAST

DESCRIPTION	QTY	PROTEINS	VEGGIES	FRUITS & NUTS	CARBS	FATS

LUNCH

DESCRIPTION	QTY	PROTEINS	VEGGIES	FRUITS & NUTS	CARBS	FATS

DINNER

DESCRIPTION	QTY	PROTEINS	VEGGIES	FRUITS & NUTS	CARBS	FATS

SNACKS

NOTES:

_____

_____

_____

_____

_____

_____

DATE:

BREAKFAST

DESCRIPTION	QTY	PROTEINS	VEGGIES	FRUITS & NUTS	CARBS	FATS

LUNCH

DESCRIPTION	QTY	PROTEINS	VEGGIES	FRUITS & NUTS	CARBS	FATS

DINNER

DESCRIPTION	QTY	PROTEINS	VEGGIES	FRUITS & NUTS	CARBS	FATS

SNACKS

NOTES:

_____

_____

_____

_____

_____

_____

DATE:

BREAKFAST

DESCRIPTION	QTY	PROTEINS	VEGGIES	FRUITS & NUTS	CARBS	FATS

LUNCH

DESCRIPTION	QTY	PROTEINS	VEGGIES	FRUITS & NUTS	CARBS	FATS

DINNER

DESCRIPTION	QTY	PROTEINS	VEGGIES	FRUITS & NUTS	CARBS	FATS

SNACKS

NOTES:

_____

_____

_____

_____

_____

_____

DATE:

BREAKFAST

DESCRIPTION	QTY	PROTEINS	VEGGIES	FRUITS & NUTS	CARBS	FATS

LUNCH

DESCRIPTION	QTY	PROTEINS	VEGGIES	FRUITS & NUTS	CARBS	FATS

DINNER

DESCRIPTION	QTY	PROTEINS	VEGGIES	FRUITS & NUTS	CARBS	FATS

SNACKS

NOTES:

_____
_____
_____
_____
_____
_____
_____

DATE:

BREAKFAST

DESCRIPTION	QTY	PROTEINS	VEGGIES	FRUITS & NUTS	CARBS	FATS

LUNCH

DESCRIPTION	QTY	PROTEINS	VEGGIES	FRUITS & NUTS	CARBS	FATS

DINNER

DESCRIPTION	QTY	PROTEINS	VEGGIES	FRUITS & NUTS	CARBS	FATS

SNACKS

NOTES:

_____

_____

_____

_____

_____

_____

DATE:

BREAKFAST

DESCRIPTION	QTY	PROTEINS	VEGGIES	FRUITS & NUTS	CARBS	FATS

LUNCH

DESCRIPTION	QTY	PROTEINS	VEGGIES	FRUITS & NUTS	CARBS	FATS

DINNER

DESCRIPTION	QTY	PROTEINS	VEGGIES	FRUITS & NUTS	CARBS	FATS

SNACKS

NOTES:

_____

_____

_____

_____

_____

_____

DATE:

BREAKFAST

DESCRIPTION	QTY	PROTEINS	VEGGIES	FRUITS & NUTS	CARBS	FATS

LUNCH

DESCRIPTION	QTY	PROTEINS	VEGGIES	FRUITS & NUTS	CARBS	FATS

DINNER

DESCRIPTION	QTY	PROTEINS	VEGGIES	FRUITS & NUTS	CARBS	FATS

SNACKS

NOTES:

DATE:

BREAKFAST

DESCRIPTION	QTY	PROTEINS	VEGGIES	FRUITS & NUTS	CARBS	FATS

LUNCH

DESCRIPTION	QTY	PROTEINS	VEGGIES	FRUITS & NUTS	CARBS	FATS

DINNER

DESCRIPTION	QTY	PROTEINS	VEGGIES	FRUITS & NUTS	CARBS	FATS

SNACKS

NOTES:

DATE:

BREAKFAST

DESCRIPTION	QTY	PROTEINS	VEGGIES	FRUITS & NUTS	CARBS	FATS

LUNCH

DESCRIPTION	QTY	PROTEINS	VEGGIES	FRUITS & NUTS	CARBS	FATS

DINNER

DESCRIPTION	QTY	PROTEINS	VEGGIES	FRUITS & NUTS	CARBS	FATS

SNACKS

NOTES:

_____

_____

_____

_____

_____

_____

DATE:

BREAKFAST

DESCRIPTION	QTY	PROTEINS	VEGGIES	FRUITS & NUTS	CARBS	FATS

LUNCH

DESCRIPTION	QTY	PROTEINS	VEGGIES	FRUITS & NUTS	CARBS	FATS

DINNER

DESCRIPTION	QTY	PROTEINS	VEGGIES	FRUITS & NUTS	CARBS	FATS

SNACKS

NOTES:

DATE:

BREAKFAST

DESCRIPTION	QTY	PROTEINS	VEGGIES	FRUITS & NUTS	CARBS	FATS

LUNCH

DESCRIPTION	QTY	PROTEINS	VEGGIES	FRUITS & NUTS	CARBS	FATS

DINNER

DESCRIPTION	QTY	PROTEINS	VEGGIES	FRUITS & NUTS	CARBS	FATS

SNACKS

NOTES:

_____

_____

_____

_____

_____

_____

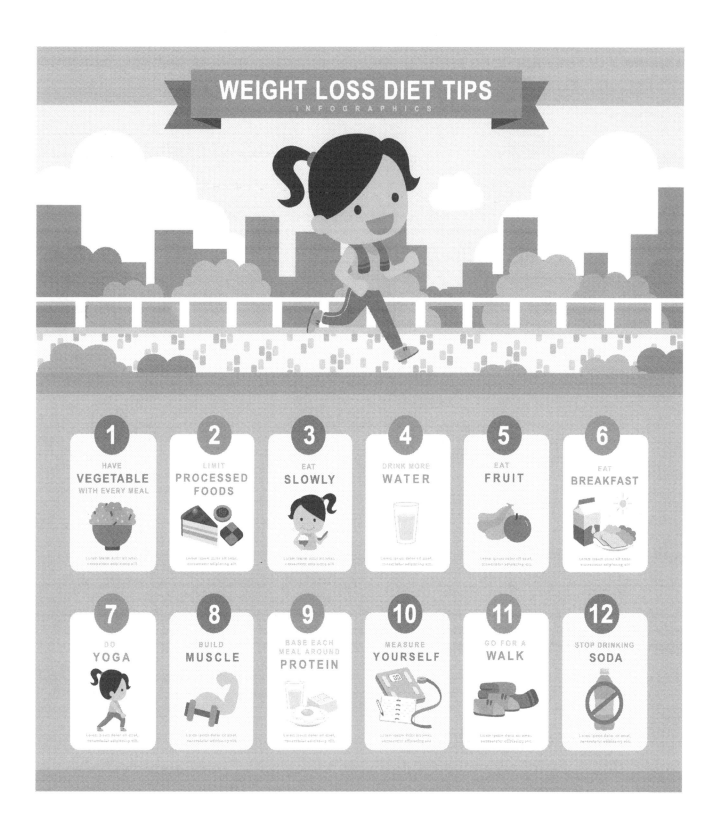

NOTES

_____

_____

_____

DATE:

BREAKFAST

DESCRIPTION	QTY	PROTEINS	VEGGIES	FRUITS & NUTS	CARBS	FATS

LUNCH

DESCRIPTION	QTY	PROTEINS	VEGGIES	FRUITS & NUTS	CARBS	FATS

DINNER

DESCRIPTION	QTY	PROTEINS	VEGGIES	FRUITS & NUTS	CARBS	FATS

SNACKS

NOTES:

_____

_____

_____

_____

_____

_____

DATE:

BREAKFAST

DESCRIPTION	QTY	PROTEINS	VEGGIES	FRUITS & NUTS	CARBS	FATS

LUNCH

DESCRIPTION	QTY	PROTEINS	VEGGIES	FRUITS & NUTS	CARBS	FATS

DINNER

DESCRIPTION	QTY	PROTEINS	VEGGIES	FRUITS & NUTS	CARBS	FATS

SNACKS

NOTES:

_____

_____

_____

_____

_____

_____

DATE:

BREAKFAST

DESCRIPTION	QTY	PROTEINS	VEGGIES	FRUITS & NUTS	CARBS	FATS

LUNCH

DESCRIPTION	QTY	PROTEINS	VEGGIES	FRUITS & NUTS	CARBS	FATS

DINNER

DESCRIPTION	QTY	PROTEINS	VEGGIES	FRUITS & NUTS	CARBS	FATS

SNACKS

NOTES:

_____

_____

_____

_____

_____

_____

DATE:

BREAKFAST

DESCRIPTION	QTY	PROTEINS	VEGGIES	FRUITS & NUTS	CARBS	FATS

LUNCH

DESCRIPTION	QTY	PROTEINS	VEGGIES	FRUITS & NUTS	CARBS	FATS

DINNER

DESCRIPTION	QTY	PROTEINS	VEGGIES	FRUITS & NUTS	CARBS	FATS

SNACKS

NOTES:

_____

_____

_____

_____

_____

_____

DATE:

BREAKFAST

DESCRIPTION	QTY	PROTEINS	VEGGIES	FRUITS & NUTS	CARBS	FATS

LUNCH

DESCRIPTION	QTY	PROTEINS	VEGGIES	FRUITS & NUTS	CARBS	FATS

DINNER

DESCRIPTION	QTY	PROTEINS	VEGGIES	FRUITS & NUTS	CARBS	FATS

SNACKS

NOTES:

_____

_____

_____

_____

_____

_____

_____

DATE:

BREAKFAST

DESCRIPTION	QTY	PROTEINS	VEGGIES	FRUITS & NUTS	CARBS	FATS

LUNCH

DESCRIPTION	QTY	PROTEINS	VEGGIES	FRUITS & NUTS	CARBS	FATS

DINNER

DESCRIPTION	QTY	PROTEINS	VEGGIES	FRUITS & NUTS	CARBS	FATS

SNACKS

NOTES:

_____

_____

_____

_____

_____

_____

DATE:

BREAKFAST

DESCRIPTION	QTY	PROTEINS	VEGGIES	FRUITS & NUTS	CARBS	FATS

LUNCH

DESCRIPTION	QTY	PROTEINS	VEGGIES	FRUITS & NUTS	CARBS	FATS

DINNER

DESCRIPTION	QTY	PROTEINS	VEGGIES	FRUITS & NUTS	CARBS	FATS

SNACKS

NOTES:

_____

_____

_____

_____

_____

_____

DATE:

BREAKFAST

DESCRIPTION	QTY	PROTEINS	VEGGIES	FRUITS & NUTS	CARBS	FATS

LUNCH

DESCRIPTION	QTY	PROTEINS	VEGGIES	FRUITS & NUTS	CARBS	FATS

DINNER

DESCRIPTION	QTY	PROTEINS	VEGGIES	FRUITS & NUTS	CARBS	FATS

SNACKS

NOTES:

DATE:

BREAKFAST

DESCRIPTION	QTY	PROTEINS	VEGGIES	FRUITS & NUTS	CARBS	FATS

LUNCH

DESCRIPTION	QTY	PROTEINS	VEGGIES	FRUITS & NUTS	CARBS	FATS

DINNER

DESCRIPTION	QTY	PROTEINS	VEGGIES	FRUITS & NUTS	CARBS	FATS

SNACKS

NOTES:

DATE:

BREAKFAST

DESCRIPTION	QTY	PROTEINS	VEGGIES	FRUITS & NUTS	CARBS	FATS

LUNCH

DESCRIPTION	QTY	PROTEINS	VEGGIES	FRUITS & NUTS	CARBS	FATS

DINNER

DESCRIPTION	QTY	PROTEINS	VEGGIES	FRUITS & NUTS	CARBS	FATS

SNACKS

NOTES:

DATE:

BREAKFAST

DESCRIPTION	QTY	PROTEINS	VEGGIES	FRUITS & NUTS	CARBS	FATS

LUNCH

DESCRIPTION	QTY	PROTEINS	VEGGIES	FRUITS & NUTS	CARBS	FATS

DINNER

DESCRIPTION	QTY	PROTEINS	VEGGIES	FRUITS & NUTS	CARBS	FATS

SNACKS

NOTES:

DATE:

BREAKFAST

DESCRIPTION	QTY	PROTEINS	VEGGIES	FRUITS & NUTS	CARBS	FATS

LUNCH

DESCRIPTION	QTY	PROTEINS	VEGGIES	FRUITS & NUTS	CARBS	FATS

DINNER

DESCRIPTION	QTY	PROTEINS	VEGGIES	FRUITS & NUTS	CARBS	FATS

SNACKS

NOTES:

DATE:

BREAKFAST

DESCRIPTION	QTY	PROTEINS	VEGGIES	FRUITS & NUTS	CARBS	FATS

LUNCH

DESCRIPTION	QTY	PROTEINS	VEGGIES	FRUITS & NUTS	CARBS	FATS

DINNER

DESCRIPTION	QTY	PROTEINS	VEGGIES	FRUITS & NUTS	CARBS	FATS

SNACKS

NOTES:

_____

_____

_____

_____

_____

_____

DATE:

BREAKFAST

DESCRIPTION	QTY	PROTEINS	VEGGIES	FRUITS & NUTS	CARBS	FATS

LUNCH

DESCRIPTION	QTY	PROTEINS	VEGGIES	FRUITS & NUTS	CARBS	FATS

DINNER

DESCRIPTION	QTY	PROTEINS	VEGGIES	FRUITS & NUTS	CARBS	FATS

SNACKS

NOTES:

_____

_____

_____

_____

_____

_____

DATE:

BREAKFAST

DESCRIPTION	QTY	PROTEINS	VEGGIES	FRUITS & NUTS	CARBS	FATS

LUNCH

DESCRIPTION	QTY	PROTEINS	VEGGIES	FRUITS & NUTS	CARBS	FATS

DINNER

DESCRIPTION	QTY	PROTEINS	VEGGIES	FRUITS & NUTS	CARBS	FATS

SNACKS

NOTES:

DATE:

BREAKFAST

DESCRIPTION	QTY	PROTEINS	VEGGIES	FRUITS & NUTS	CARBS	FATS

LUNCH

DESCRIPTION	QTY	PROTEINS	VEGGIES	FRUITS & NUTS	CARBS	FATS

DINNER

DESCRIPTION	QTY	PROTEINS	VEGGIES	FRUITS & NUTS	CARBS	FATS

SNACKS

NOTES:

_____

_____

_____

_____

_____

_____

DATE:

BREAKFAST

DESCRIPTION	QTY	PROTEINS	VEGGIES	FRUITS & NUTS	CARBS	FATS

LUNCH

DESCRIPTION	QTY	PROTEINS	VEGGIES	FRUITS & NUTS	CARBS	FATS

DINNER

DESCRIPTION	QTY	PROTEINS	VEGGIES	FRUITS & NUTS	CARBS	FATS

SNACKS

NOTES:

DATE:

BREAKFAST

DESCRIPTION	QTY	PROTEINS	VEGGIES	FRUITS & NUTS	CARBS	FATS

LUNCH

DESCRIPTION	QTY	PROTEINS	VEGGIES	FRUITS & NUTS	CARBS	FATS

DINNER

DESCRIPTION	QTY	PROTEINS	VEGGIES	FRUITS & NUTS	CARBS	FATS

SNACKS

NOTES:

_____

_____

_____

_____

_____

_____

DATE:

BREAKFAST

DESCRIPTION	QTY	PROTEINS	VEGGIES	FRUITS & NUTS	CARBS	FATS

LUNCH

DESCRIPTION	QTY	PROTEINS	VEGGIES	FRUITS & NUTS	CARBS	FATS

DINNER

DESCRIPTION	QTY	PROTEINS	VEGGIES	FRUITS & NUTS	CARBS	FATS

SNACKS

NOTES:

DATE:

BREAKFAST

DESCRIPTION	QTY	PROTEINS	VEGGIES	FRUITS & NUTS	CARBS	FATS

LUNCH

DESCRIPTION	QTY	PROTEINS	VEGGIES	FRUITS & NUTS	CARBS	FATS

DINNER

DESCRIPTION	QTY	PROTEINS	VEGGIES	FRUITS & NUTS	CARBS	FATS

SNACKS

NOTES:

_____

_____

_____

_____

_____

_____

DATE:

BREAKFAST

DESCRIPTION	QTY	PROTEINS	VEGGIES	FRUITS & NUTS	CARBS	FATS

LUNCH

DESCRIPTION	QTY	PROTEINS	VEGGIES	FRUITS & NUTS	CARBS	FATS

DINNER

DESCRIPTION	QTY	PROTEINS	VEGGIES	FRUITS & NUTS	CARBS	FATS

SNACKS

NOTES:

_____

_____

_____

_____

_____

_____

DATE:

BREAKFAST

DESCRIPTION	QTY	PROTEINS	VEGGIES	FRUITS & NUTS	CARBS	FATS

LUNCH

DESCRIPTION	QTY	PROTEINS	VEGGIES	FRUITS & NUTS	CARBS	FATS

DINNER

DESCRIPTION	QTY	PROTEINS	VEGGIES	FRUITS & NUTS	CARBS	FATS

SNACKS

NOTES:

_____

_____

_____

_____

_____

_____

DATE:

BREAKFAST

DESCRIPTION	QTY	PROTEINS	VEGGIES	FRUITS & NUTS	CARBS	FATS

LUNCH

DESCRIPTION	QTY	PROTEINS	VEGGIES	FRUITS & NUTS	CARBS	FATS

DINNER

DESCRIPTION	QTY	PROTEINS	VEGGIES	FRUITS & NUTS	CARBS	FATS

SNACKS

NOTES:

_____

_____

_____

_____

_____

_____

DATE:

BREAKFAST

DESCRIPTION	QTY	PROTEINS	VEGGIES	FRUITS & NUTS	CARBS	FATS

LUNCH

DESCRIPTION	QTY	PROTEINS	VEGGIES	FRUITS & NUTS	CARBS	FATS

DINNER

DESCRIPTION	QTY	PROTEINS	VEGGIES	FRUITS & NUTS	CARBS	FATS

SNACKS

NOTES:

DATE:

BREAKFAST

DESCRIPTION	QTY	PROTEINS	VEGGIES	FRUITS & NUTS	CARBS	FATS

LUNCH

DESCRIPTION	QTY	PROTEINS	VEGGIES	FRUITS & NUTS	CARBS	FATS

DINNER

DESCRIPTION	QTY	PROTEINS	VEGGIES	FRUITS & NUTS	CARBS	FATS

SNACKS

NOTES:

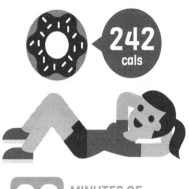

242 cals

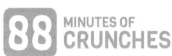

88 MINUTES OF CRUNCHES

THINK
— BEFORE —
YOU EAT

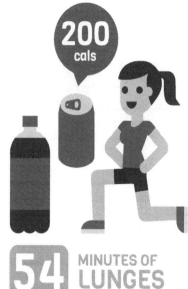

200 cals

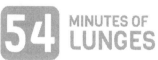

54 MINUTES OF LUNGES

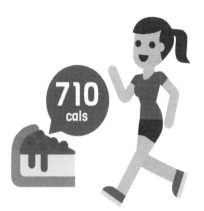

710 cals

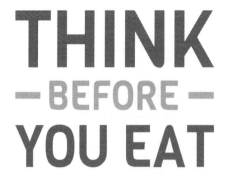

444 cals

FRIED CHICKEN BREAST

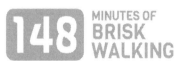

148 MINUTES OF BRISK WALKING

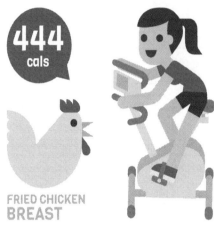

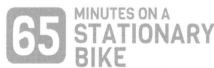

65 MINUTES ON A STATIONARY BIKE

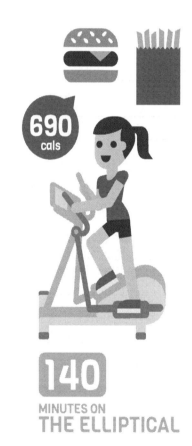

690 cals

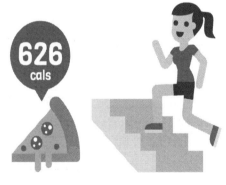

626 cals

MILKSHAKE

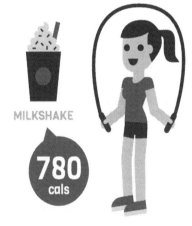

780 cals

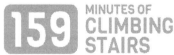

159 MINUTES OF CLIMBING STAIRS

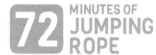

72 MINUTES OF JUMPING ROPE

140 MINUTES ON THE ELLIPTICAL

MY THOUGHTS:

_____

_____

_____

DATE:

BREAKFAST

DESCRIPTION	QTY	PROTEINS	VEGGIES	FRUITS & NUTS	CARBS	FATS

LUNCH

DESCRIPTION	QTY	PROTEINS	VEGGIES	FRUITS & NUTS	CARBS	FATS

DINNER

DESCRIPTION	QTY	PROTEINS	VEGGIES	FRUITS & NUTS	CARBS	FATS

SNACKS

NOTES:

_____

_____

_____

_____

_____

_____

DATE:

BREAKFAST

DESCRIPTION	QTY	PROTEINS	VEGGIES	FRUITS & NUTS	CARBS	FATS

LUNCH

DESCRIPTION	QTY	PROTEINS	VEGGIES	FRUITS & NUTS	CARBS	FATS

DINNER

DESCRIPTION	QTY	PROTEINS	VEGGIES	FRUITS & NUTS	CARBS	FATS

SNACKS

NOTES:

_____

_____

_____

_____

_____

_____

DATE:

BREAKFAST

DESCRIPTION	QTY	PROTEINS	VEGGIES	FRUITS & NUTS	CARBS	FATS

LUNCH

DESCRIPTION	QTY	PROTEINS	VEGGIES	FRUITS & NUTS	CARBS	FATS

DINNER

DESCRIPTION	QTY	PROTEINS	VEGGIES	FRUITS & NUTS	CARBS	FATS

SNACKS

NOTES:

DATE:

BREAKFAST

DESCRIPTION	QTY	PROTEINS	VEGGIES	FRUITS & NUTS	CARBS	FATS

LUNCH

DESCRIPTION	QTY	PROTEINS	VEGGIES	FRUITS & NUTS	CARBS	FATS

DINNER

DESCRIPTION	QTY	PROTEINS	VEGGIES	FRUITS & NUTS	CARBS	FATS

SNACKS

NOTES:

DATE:

BREAKFAST

DESCRIPTION	QTY	PROTEINS	VEGGIES	FRUITS & NUTS	CARBS	FATS

LUNCH

DESCRIPTION	QTY	PROTEINS	VEGGIES	FRUITS & NUTS	CARBS	FATS

DINNER

DESCRIPTION	QTY	PROTEINS	VEGGIES	FRUITS & NUTS	CARBS	FATS

SNACKS

NOTES:

DATE:

BREAKFAST

DESCRIPTION	QTY	PROTEINS	VEGGIES	FRUITS & NUTS	CARBS	FATS

LUNCH

DESCRIPTION	QTY	PROTEINS	VEGGIES	FRUITS & NUTS	CARBS	FATS

DINNER

DESCRIPTION	QTY	PROTEINS	VEGGIES	FRUITS & NUTS	CARBS	FATS

SNACKS

NOTES:

_____

_____

_____

_____

_____

_____

DATE:

BREAKFAST

DESCRIPTION	QTY	PROTEINS	VEGGIES	FRUITS & NUTS	CARBS	FATS

LUNCH

DESCRIPTION	QTY	PROTEINS	VEGGIES	FRUITS & NUTS	CARBS	FATS

DINNER

DESCRIPTION	QTY	PROTEINS	VEGGIES	FRUITS & NUTS	CARBS	FATS

SNACKS

NOTES:

_____

_____

_____

_____

_____

_____

_____

DATE:

BREAKFAST

DESCRIPTION	QTY	PROTEINS	VEGGIES	FRUITS & NUTS	CARBS	FATS

LUNCH

DESCRIPTION	QTY	PROTEINS	VEGGIES	FRUITS & NUTS	CARBS	FATS

DINNER

DESCRIPTION	QTY	PROTEINS	VEGGIES	FRUITS & NUTS	CARBS	FATS

SNACKS

NOTES:

DATE:

BREAKFAST

DESCRIPTION	QTY	PROTEINS	VEGGIES	FRUITS & NUTS	CARBS	FATS

LUNCH

DESCRIPTION	QTY	PROTEINS	VEGGIES	FRUITS & NUTS	CARBS	FATS

DINNER

DESCRIPTION	QTY	PROTEINS	VEGGIES	FRUITS & NUTS	CARBS	FATS

SNACKS

NOTES:

DATE:

BREAKFAST

DESCRIPTION	QTY	PROTEINS	VEGGIES	FRUITS & NUTS	CARBS	FATS

LUNCH

DESCRIPTION	QTY	PROTEINS	VEGGIES	FRUITS & NUTS	CARBS	FATS

DINNER

DESCRIPTION	QTY	PROTEINS	VEGGIES	FRUITS & NUTS	CARBS	FATS

SNACKS

NOTES:

_____

_____

_____

_____

_____

_____

DATE:

BREAKFAST

DESCRIPTION	QTY	PROTEINS	VEGGIES	FRUITS & NUTS	CARBS	FATS

LUNCH

DESCRIPTION	QTY	PROTEINS	VEGGIES	FRUITS & NUTS	CARBS	FATS

DINNER

DESCRIPTION	QTY	PROTEINS	VEGGIES	FRUITS & NUTS	CARBS	FATS

SNACKS

NOTES:

_____

_____

_____

_____

_____

_____

DATE:

BREAKFAST

DESCRIPTION	QTY	PROTEINS	VEGGIES	FRUITS & NUTS	CARBS	FATS

LUNCH

DESCRIPTION	QTY	PROTEINS	VEGGIES	FRUITS & NUTS	CARBS	FATS

DINNER

DESCRIPTION	QTY	PROTEINS	VEGGIES	FRUITS & NUTS	CARBS	FATS

SNACKS

NOTES:

DATE:

BREAKFAST

DESCRIPTION	QTY	PROTEINS	VEGGIES	FRUITS & NUTS	CARBS	FATS

LUNCH

DESCRIPTION	QTY	PROTEINS	VEGGIES	FRUITS & NUTS	CARBS	FATS

DINNER

DESCRIPTION	QTY	PROTEINS	VEGGIES	FRUITS & NUTS	CARBS	FATS

SNACKS

NOTES:

DATE:

BREAKFAST

DESCRIPTION	QTY	PROTEINS	VEGGIES	FRUITS & NUTS	CARBS	FATS

LUNCH

DESCRIPTION	QTY	PROTEINS	VEGGIES	FRUITS & NUTS	CARBS	FATS

DINNER

DESCRIPTION	QTY	PROTEINS	VEGGIES	FRUITS & NUTS	CARBS	FATS

SNACKS

NOTES:

_____

_____

_____

_____

_____

_____